THE 30-MINUTE GLUTEN-FREE VEGAN COOKBOOK FOR BEGINNERS

150 simple, Nutritious and Delicious plant-base recipes for beginners

AVILA WANDA

THE 30-MINUTE GLUTEN-FREE VEGAN COOKBOOK FOR BEGINNERS

Introduction

In the bustling heart of the city, where time seemed to race faster than ever, lived Avila—a passionate food enthusiast with a mission. As a firm believer in the power of nourishing, plant-based meals, Avila embarked on a journey to demystify the seemingly complex world of gluten-free vegan cooking. Her inspiration? A desire to make wholesome, delicious meals accessible to everyone, even in the midst of hectic schedules.

Avila's culinary adventure began when she faced the challenge of accommodating her friend's dietary restrictions. Determined to create dishes that were not only inclusive but also quick and simple, she dove headfirst into the art of gluten-free vegan cooking. The result of her exploration? The "30-Minute Gluten-Free Vegan Cookbook for Beginners."

The cookbook became Avila's labor of love, crafted for those who yearned for a delectable escape from the mundane, without compromising their health or values. Each recipe was a testament to her dedication—meticulously designed to transform humble ingredients into culinary delights in half an hour or less.

Within the pages of her cookbook, Avila wove a narrative of flavors, textures, and colors that danced harmoniously on the plate. From hearty quinoa salads to savory chickpea stews, she curated a collection of recipes that not only satisfied the palate but also celebrated the vibrant world of plant-based ingredients.

Avila's mission extended beyond providing mere recipes; she sought to empower beginners on their gluten-free vegan journey. The introductory section of her cookbook served as a guiding light, offering insights into essential pantry staples, cooking techniques, and time-saving tips. As readers flipped through the pages, they discovered the joy of preparing meals that embraced both health and taste—a perfect union of mindful eating and culinary delight.

The 30-minute promise was more than a convenience; it was a declaration that wholesome, plant-based cooking need not be a time-consuming affair. Avila's cookbook became a trusted companion for those navigating the realms of gluten-free veganism, proving that delicious, nutritious meals were within reach, even on the busiest of days.

In the heart of Avila's culinary haven, where simplicity met sophistication, the "30-Minute Gluten-Free Vegan Cookbook for Beginners" emerged as a beacon, guiding individuals toward a flavorful, compassionate, and time-efficient approach to nourishing their bodies and souls.

Chapter one

Gluten and it's resistance

Gluten, a complex mixture of proteins found in wheat and related grains, plays a crucial role in determining the unique texture and structure of baked goods. However, for some individuals, gluten can pose health challenges due to conditions like celiac disease, wheat allergy, or non-celiac gluten sensitivity.

1. Celiac Disease:
   - *Overview:* Celiac disease is an autoimmune disorder where the ingestion of gluten triggers an immune response, damaging the small intestine lining.
   - *Genetic Factors:* It has a strong genetic component, and

individuals with specific genetic markers are more susceptible.

- *Symptoms:* Digestive issues, fatigue, weight loss, and nutrient deficiencies are common symptoms.
- *Diagnosis:* Typically confirmed through blood tests measuring specific antibodies and confirmed with a small intestinal biopsy.

2. Wheat Allergy:

- *Overview:* Wheat allergy is an immune response to proteins in wheat, including but not limited to gluten.
- *Symptoms:* Allergic reactions can range from mild to severe, involving hives, digestive issues,

difficulty breathing, and in
extreme cases, anaphylaxis.

- *Diagnosis:* Skin tests, blood tests, and food challenges may be used for diagnosis.

3. Non-Celiac Gluten Sensitivity (NCGS):
   - *Overview:* Unlike celiac disease and wheat allergy, NCGS is not an autoimmune or allergic reaction but an adverse reaction to gluten.
   - *Symptoms:* NCGS can present with symptoms similar to celiac disease but without the autoimmune component.
   - *Diagnosis:* It is a diagnosis of exclusion, meaning other conditions are ruled out, and

symptoms improve on a gluten-free diet.

4. Gluten Resistance:

- *Definition:* The term "gluten resistance" is not a recognized medical condition. If referring to difficulty digesting gluten or experiencing symptoms despite a gluten-free diet, it may align more closely with NCGS.
- *Potential Causes:* Some individuals may experience persistent symptoms due to cross-contamination, inadvertent gluten exposure, or sensitivity to other components in gluten-containing grains.

5. Managing Gluten-Related Conditions:

- *Gluten-Free Diet:* The primary treatment for celiac disease and wheat allergy is a strict gluten-free diet, eliminating wheat and gluten-containing grains.

- *Nutritional Considerations:* Individuals on a gluten-free diet must pay attention to nutritional deficiencies, as some essential nutrients may be lacking.

- *Ongoing Research:* The understanding of gluten-related conditions is evolving, with ongoing research exploring potential therapies and diagnostic methods.

Challenges for being a gluten resistance

1. Dietary Restrictions:

   Keeping up a gluten-free diet may be difficult since gluten can be found in a lot of everyday items.Reading labels and being vigilant about cross-contamination becomes a daily concern.

2. Social and Lifestyle Impact:

   Following a gluten-free diet may affect social interactions, dining out, and participating in certain events where gluten-containing foods are prevalent.

3. Nutritional Concerns:

Gluten-free diets might be low in certain nutrients like fiber, B vitamins, and iron if not carefully planned. Individuals may need to find alternative sources or consider supplements.

4. Expense:

Gluten-free specialty products can be more expensive than their gluten-containing counterparts, potentially leading to increased grocery bills.

5. Emotional Impact:

Adapting to a gluten-free lifestyle can
bring emotional challenges, including
frustration, anxiety, or feelings of
isolation, especially in social situations
involving food.

6. Diagnosis Delays:

Some individuals may experience
delays in receiving a proper diagnosis
due to a lack of awareness about
gluten-related conditions or variations in
symptoms.

7. Hidden Gluten:

Gluten can be present in unexpected places, such as sauces, condiments, and processed foods, making it challenging to avoid entirely.

8. Cross-Contamination:

Avoiding cross-contamination in shared kitchens or dining spaces can be difficult, and accidental exposure to gluten can lead to symptoms for those with gluten sensitivity or celiac disease.

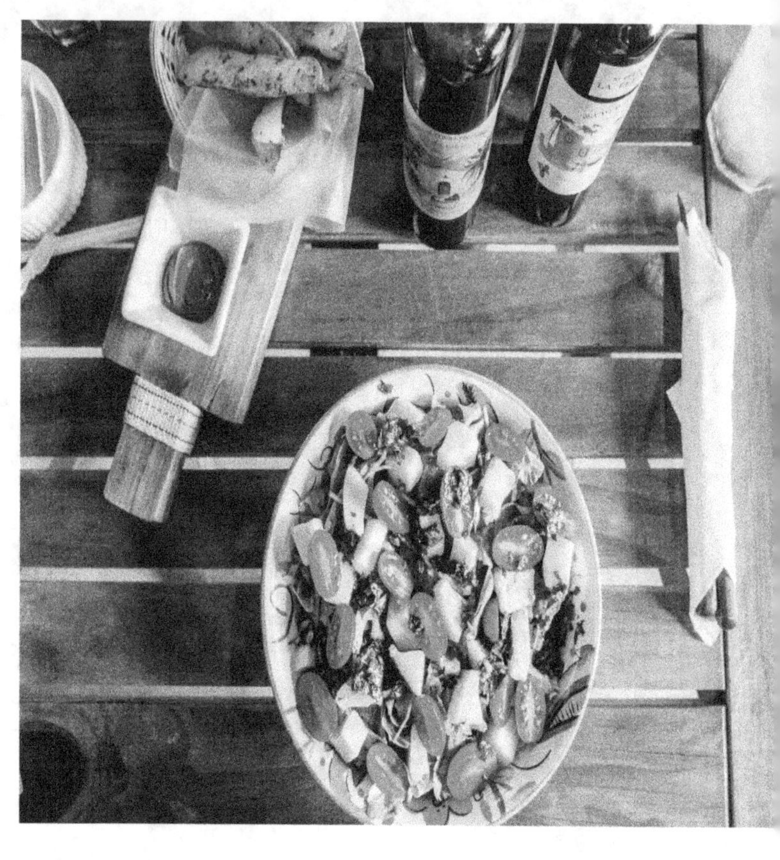

Chapter two

Challengs of Celiac diseases

Living with celiac disease, an autoimmune disorder triggered by the ingestion of gluten, poses several challenges. Here are some key difficulties associated with celiac disease:

1. Strict Dietary Restrictions:

   Managing celiac disease necessitates a strict, lifelong adherence to a gluten-free diet. Gluten is found in many common foods, and avoiding it requires careful reading of labels and awareness of potential cross-contamination.

2. Social and Dining Challenges:

Social situations and dining out can be
challenging due to limited gluten-free
options, potential cross-contamination
risks, and the need to communicate
dietary restrictions to others.

3. Emotional Impact:

Adapting to a gluten-free lifestyle can be
emotionally challenging. Feelings of
frustration, isolation, and anxiety about
accidental gluten exposure are
common.

4. Medical Monitoring:

Regular medical check-ups and monitoring are essential to assess the impact of celiac disease on the body, including potential nutritional deficiencies and associated health conditions.

5. Cross-Contamination Concerns:

Preventing cross-contamination in shared kitchens or dining spaces is a constant concern. Individuals with celiac disease must be vigilant about cooking utensils, cutting boards, and other potential sources of gluten.

6. Nutritional Deficiencies:

Celiac disease can lead to nutrient

malabsorption, resulting in deficiencies

in vitamins and minerals such as iron,

calcium, and B vitamins. Nutritional

supplementation or dietary adjustments

may be necessary.

7. Limited Food Options:

Finding suitable gluten-free alternatives,

especially for processed foods, can be

challenging. Gluten-free specialty

products may also be more expensive.

8. Delayed Diagnosis:

Some individuals may experience delays in receiving a proper diagnosis due to varied and sometimes subtle symptoms, which can impact their overall health.

9. Increased Risk of Other Conditions:

Untreated or poorly managed celiac disease can increase the risk of developing other autoimmune disorders, osteoporosis, infertility, and certain cancers.

10.   Travel Challenges:

Traveling, especially to regions with limited gluten-free options or varying levels of awareness about celiac disease, can be challenging. Planning and communication are crucial.

Challenges of non-celiac gluten sensitivity

Non-celiac gluten sensitivity (NCGS) poses several challenges, including:

1. Diagnosis Difficulties: Unlike celiac disease, there is no specific diagnostic test for NCGS. Diagnosis often relies on the exclusion of other conditions,

making it challenging to identify
definitively.

2. Symptom Variability: Symptoms of
   NCGS can vary widely and may overlap
   with other gastrointestinal disorders,
   making it challenging to attribute them
   solely to gluten sensitivity.

3. Lack of Biomarkers: Unlike celiac
   disease, there are no specific
   biomarkers for NCGS. This absence of
   objective markers makes it difficult to
   measure and monitor the condition
   objectively.

4. Controversial Nature: The existence and
   characterization of NCGS are still
   debated within the medical community.
   Some argue that it might be a spectrum
   of disorders rather than a distinct entity.

5. Dietary Restrictions: Managing NCGS requires strict adherence to a gluten-free diet, which can be challenging due to the ubiquity of gluten in many food products.

6. Psychosocial Impact: Following a gluten-free diet can have social and psychological implications, affecting one's lifestyle and social interactions.

7. Research Gaps: There is a lack of comprehensive research on NCGS, including its prevalence, underlying mechanisms, and long-term effects. This hinders the development of effective treatments.

Challenges of Wheat Allergy

Wheat allergy presents several challenges, including:

1. Immediate Allergic Reactions: Wheat allergy can lead to immediate allergic reactions, such as hives, swelling, and anaphylaxis. Managing these reactions requires prompt and often emergency medical intervention.

2. Cross-Reactivity: Individuals with wheat allergy may experience cross-reactivity with other grains or foods, complicating dietary restrictions.

3. Hidden Wheat Ingredients: Identifying and avoiding wheat in food products can be challenging due to its presence in

various forms and as a hidden ingredient in processed foods.

4. Bread and Staple Food Elimination: Wheat is a staple in many diets, and eliminating it can be difficult, leading to potential nutritional deficiencies.

5. Impact on Social Interactions: Managing a wheat allergy may impact social activities, dining out, and attending events where food is served, making it challenging to navigate social situations.

6. Labeling Issues: Inconsistent or unclear food labeling can make it difficult for individuals with wheat allergy to confidently choose safe products.

7. Limited Treatment Options: Unlike some other allergies, there is currently no specific medication for treating wheat allergy. Management relies on

avoidance and, in case of accidental
exposure, prompt use of epinephrine.

8. Outgrowing Uncertainty: Wheat allergy
    is more common in children, and while
    some may outgrow it, the uncertainty of
    when or if this will happen can be
    challenging for both patients and their
    families.

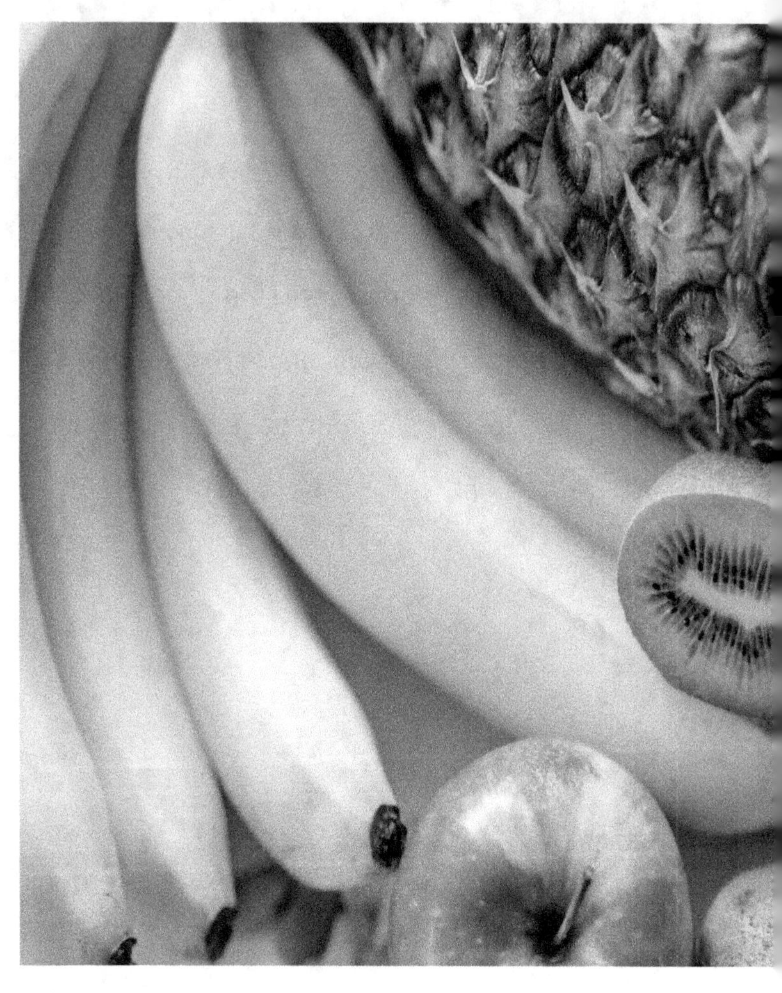

Chapter three

What does gluten do

Gluten serves several crucial functions in baking and cooking due to its unique properties:

1. Structural Integrity:

    ○ *Protein Network:* Gluten forms a protein network when mixed with water, creating a structural framework that traps carbon dioxide produced during fermentation or leavening. This gives bread and other baked goods their characteristic rise and texture.

2. Texture and Elasticity:

   - *Stretchiness:* Gluten provides elasticity to dough, allowing it to stretch and expand without breaking. This contributes to the chewy texture in bread and the structure in pasta.

3. Volume and Fluffiness:

   - *Leavening Agent:* As yeast ferments and produces carbon dioxide, gluten captures and holds these gas bubbles. This results in the expansion of the dough, contributing to the volume and fluffiness of baked goods.

4. Moisture Retention:

   - *Water Binding:* Gluten has water-binding properties, helping to retain moisture in the dough or batter. This contributes to the softness and freshness of baked products.

5. Tenderizing Effect:

   - *Starch Interaction:* Gluten interacts with starch molecules, preventing them from forming a rigid structure. This tenderizing effect is particularly important in certain baked goods like cakes and pastries.

While gluten plays a crucial role in creating desirable textures and structures in many traditional baked items, it's important to note that some individuals must avoid gluten due to health reasons, such as celiac disease, wheat allergy, or non-celiac gluten sensitivity. For them, gluten can trigger adverse reactions, and adopting a gluten-free diet is necessary for maintaining their health and well-being.

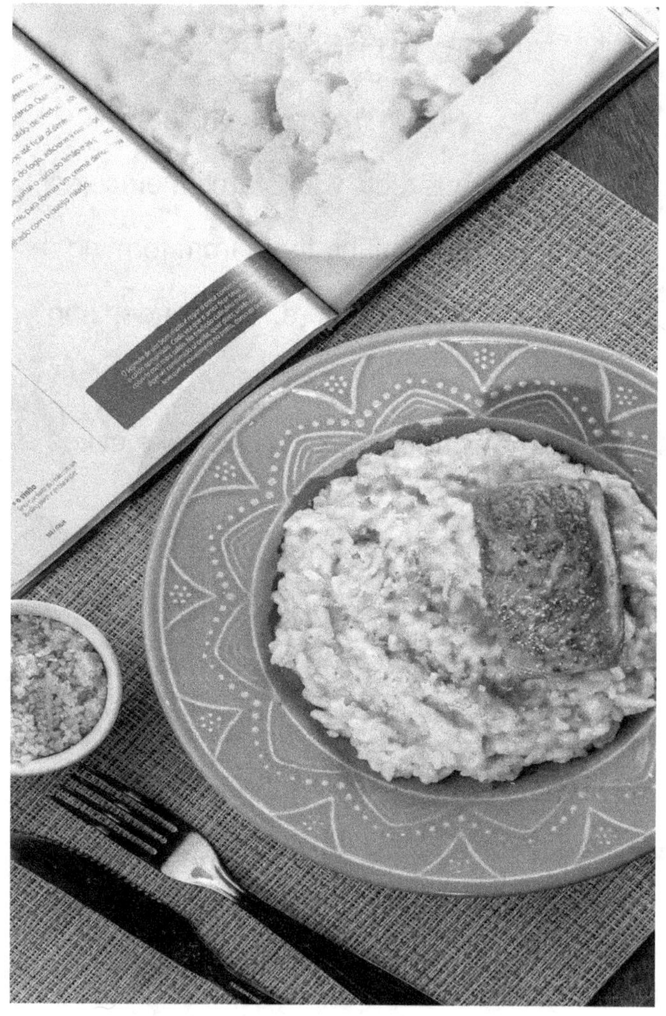

Chapter four

Vegans and it's benefits in relation with weight loss

Adopting a vegan lifestyle, which involves abstaining from the consumption of animal products, can have several potential benefits in relation to weight loss. It's important to note that individual responses to a vegan diet may vary, and factors such as overall dietary choices, portion control, and lifestyle play crucial roles. Here are some ways in which a vegan diet may contribute to weight loss:

1. Low-Calorie Density:

   - *Plant-Based Foods:* A vegan diet is often rich in whole, plant-based foods such as fruits, vegetables, legumes, and whole grains. These foods tend to have lower calorie density, allowing individuals to consume larger volumes of food for fewer calories, promoting a feeling of fullness.

2. High Fiber Content:

   - *Satiety and Digestion:* Plant-based diets are typically high in dietary fiber, which enhances satiety and promotes better digestion. Fiber-rich foods can help control appetite, reduce overeating, and contribute to weight management.

3. Nutrient-Dense Choices:

   - *Vitamins and Minerals:* A well-balanced vegan diet can

provide essential vitamins and minerals while being lower in saturated fats and cholesterol. Nutrient-dense foods support overall health and can contribute to weight loss by promoting optimal bodily functions.

4. Reduced Processed Foods:

   o *Minimized Junk Foods:* Vegan diets often encourage the consumption of whole, minimally processed foods. By minimizing the intake of highly processed and calorie-dense foods, individuals may find it easier to maintain or lose weight.

5. Plant-Based Protein Sources:

   o *Lean Protein Options:* While some animal products are rich

sources of protein, plant-based
alternatives like legumes, tofu,
tempeh, and seitan can provide
ample protein with lower
saturated fat content. Protein is
crucial for maintaining muscle
mass, which can contribute to a
healthy weight.

6. Lower Caloric Intake:

   - *Mindful Eating:* People on a
     vegan diet may become more
     mindful of their food choices,
     leading to a reduction in overall
     caloric intake. Choosing
     nutrient-dense foods over
     calorie-dense options can
     contribute to weight loss.

7. Potential Metabolic Effects:

   o *Improvements in Metabolism:* Some studies suggest that a vegan diet may have positive effects on metabolism, potentially leading to better weight management. However, individual responses can vary.

8. Increased Physical Activity:

   o *Lifestyle Choices:* Embracing a vegan lifestyle often goes hand in hand with an emphasis on holistic well-being. Many vegans adopt active lifestyles, including regular exercise, which contributes to weight loss and overall health.

While a vegan diet has potential benefits for weight loss, it's essential to approach dietary

changes with balance and mindfulness.
Consulting with a healthcare professional or a
registered dietitian can provide personalized
guidance to ensure that nutritional needs are
met while working toward weight management
goals on a vegan diet.

Vegans and vegetarians

Vegans and vegetarians are individuals who choose plant-based diets for various reasons, but they differ in the extent of their dietary restrictions. Understanding the distinctions between these two dietary lifestyles helps shed light on their motivations, dietary choices, and impact on personal health and the environment.

Vegetarians:

- *Definition:* Vegetarians abstain from consuming meat, poultry, and seafood.
- *Inclusion of Animal Products:* Many vegetarians include dairy products and eggs in their diet, depending on the

specific type of vegetarianism they follow.

* *Motivations:* Reasons for choosing a vegetarian lifestyle may include ethical concerns about animal welfare, religious beliefs, or health considerations.

Vegans:

* *Definition:* Vegans take their dietary choices a step further by excluding all animal products from their diet.
* *Complete Exclusion:* In addition to avoiding meat, vegans exclude dairy, eggs, and other animal-derived ingredients from their meals and often extend their lifestyle choices beyond diet to exclude other animal-based products like leather and honey.

- *Motivations:* Veganism is often motivated by a combination of ethical, environmental, and health concerns. Vegans aim to minimize their impact on animal exploitation, reduce environmental harm, and adopt a plant-based diet for potential health benefits.

Shared Principles:

- *Plant-Based Focus:* Both vegans and vegetarians emphasize a plant-based diet, centering their meals around fruits, vegetables, grains, legumes, nuts, and seeds.
- *Health Benefits:* Both lifestyles can provide health benefits, such as lower risks of certain diseases and conditions,

including heart disease and high blood
pressure.

Considerations:

- *Nutrient Intake:* Both vegans and
  vegetarians need to pay attention to
  certain nutrients that are more abundant
  in animal products, such as vitamin B12,
  iron, and omega-3 fatty acids.
  Supplementation or careful food choices
  can address these concerns.
- *Variability:* There is a spectrum within
  both groups, with some vegetarians
  allowing for more flexibility in their diets
  (e.g., lacto-vegetarians including dairy)
  and some vegans adopting stricter
  practices (e.g., avoiding processed

foods with hidden animal-derived ingredients).

Ultimately, whether one chooses a vegetarian or vegan lifestyle, both dietary choices have the potential to promote health and contribute to environmental sustainability. The decision often reflects an individual's personal beliefs, values, and the extent to which they are willing to abstain from various animal products.

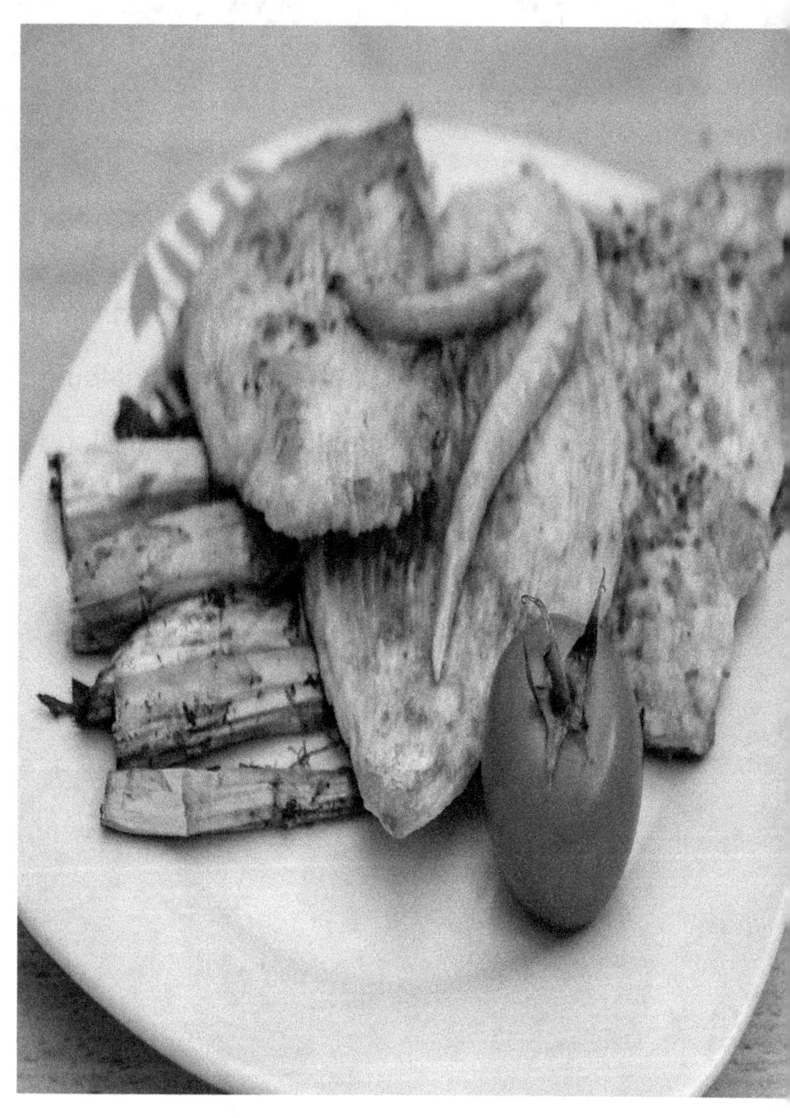

Chapter five

Delicious, quick and easy breakfast dinner recipes for glute-free vegans cookbook for beginners

Quinoa Breakfast Bowl:

1. Combine cooked quinoa with fresh berries, chopped nuts, and a drizzle of maple syrup for a hearty and nutritious gluten-free vegan breakfast.

Avocado Toast with a Twist:

2. Upgrade your classic avocado toast by adding cherry tomatoes, arugula, and a sprinkle of hemp seeds on top of gluten-free bread.

Chia Pudding Parfait:

3. Layer chia pudding with coconut yogurt and your favorite fruits in a glass for a delightful and simple gluten-free vegan breakfast.

Sweet Potato Hash:

4. Sauté diced sweet potatoes with bell peppers, onions, and black beans. Top with avocado slices for a filling and delicious breakfast hash.

Smoothie Bowl Delight:

5. Blend frozen berries, banana, spinach, and almond milk. Pour into a bowl and top with gluten-free granola, sliced almonds, and shredded coconut.

Tofu Scramble Wrap:

6. Sauté tofu with veggies like bell
    peppers, spinach, and cherry tomatoes.
    Wrap in a gluten-free tortilla for a
    satisfying breakfast on the go.

Buckwheat Pancakes:

7. Make fluffy pancakes using buckwheat
    flour. Top with fresh fruit and a dollop of
    dairy-free yogurt for a gluten-free vegan
    breakfast treat.

Coconut Rice Pudding:

8. Cook rice in coconut milk and sweeten
    with a touch of agave syrup. Serve
    warm, topped with mango slices and a
    sprinkle of toasted coconut.

Millet Porridge:

9. Cook millet with almond milk and cinnamon. Top with sliced bananas, chopped nuts, and a drizzle of date syrup for a comforting gluten-free vegan porridge.

Almond Butter and Banana Toast:

10. Spread almond butter on gluten-free toast and add banana slices. Sprinkle with chia seeds for an easy and delicious breakfast option.

Remember to adapt these recipes based on personal preferences and dietary needs. Enjoy your gluten-free vegan breakfasts!

Delicious, quick and easy lunch recipes for a glute-free vegans cookbook

Certainly! Here are some delicious, quick, and easy lunch recipes for a gluten-free vegan cookbook:

Chickpea and Vegetable Stir-Fry:

1. Sauté chickpeas with a colorful mix of broccoli, bell peppers, and snap peas. Add gluten-free tamari sauce for flavor and serve over rice or quinoa.

Mango Avocado Salad:

2. Combine diced mango, avocado, cherry tomatoes, and red onion. Toss with a simple dressing made of lime juice, olive oil, salt, and pepper.

Lentil Lettuce Wraps:

3. Cook lentils with cumin and paprika. Fill lettuce leaves with the lentil mixture, top with diced tomatoes, and drizzle with dairy-free tzatziki.

Spaghetti with Vegan Pesto:

4. Cook gluten-free spaghetti and toss with a homemade vegan pesto made from

fresh basil, pine nuts, garlic, nutritional
yeast, and olive oil.

Mexican Quinoa Bowl:

5.   Add salsa, black beans, corn, and
avocado to cooked quinoa.Top with
cilantro and a squeeze of lime for a
quick and flavorful bowl.

Crispy Tofu Salad:

6. Bake tofu until crispy and place it on a
bed of mixed greens. Add cucumber,
radishes, and a tangy vinaigrette
dressing.

Stuffed Bell Peppers:

7. Fill halved bell peppers with a mixture of quinoa, black beans, corn, and diced tomatoes. Bake until peppers are tender.

Cauliflower and Chickpea Tacos:

8. Roast cauliflower and chickpeas with taco seasoning. Fill gluten-free corn tortillas and top with shredded lettuce, salsa, and guacamole.

Mushroom and Spinach Quesadillas:

9. Sauté mushrooms and spinach, then sandwich them between gluten-free

tortillas with vegan cheese. Grill until the tortillas are golden and crispy.

Greek Salad with Quinoa:

10. Combine cooked quinoa with cucumber, cherry tomatoes, Kalamata olives, red onion, and vegan feta. Use lemon juice and olive oil to dress.

Remember to adjust these recipes based on your preferences and dietary needs. Enjoy your delicious gluten-free vegan lunches!

Delicious, quick and easy dinner recipes for glute-free vegans cookbook

Certainly! Here are some delicious, quick, and easy dinner recipes for a gluten-free vegan cookbook tailored for beginners:

Chickpea and Vegetable Curry:

1. Simmer chickpeas with a medley of colorful vegetables in a coconut milk-based curry sauce. Serve over gluten-free rice or quinoa.

Stuffed Bell Peppers with Quinoa:

2. Fill bell peppers with a mixture of cooked quinoa, black beans, corn, and spices. Bake until peppers are tender, and top with avocado.

Vegan Stir-Fried Rice:

3. Sauté a mix of vegetables like peas, carrots, and broccoli with gluten-free tamari. Add cooked rice and stir-fry for a quick and flavorful dinner.

Eggplant and Tomato Bake:

4. Arrange the tomatoes and eggplant slices in a baking dish. Drizzle with olive

oil, sprinkle with herbs, and bake until golden and tender.

Sweet Potato and Lentil Stew:

5. Combine sweet potatoes, lentils, and diced tomatoes in a pot with vegetable broth and spices. Simmer until everything is tender and flavorful.

Crispy Baked Tofu Bowl:

6. Coat tofu cubes in your favorite gluten-free seasoning and bake until crispy. Serve over a bed of quinoa with sautéed vegetables.

Zucchini Noodles with Pesto:

7. Spiralize zucchini into noodles and toss with a homemade vegan pesto made from basil, nuts, garlic, and nutritional yeast.

Mushroom and Spinach Risotto:

8. Sauté mushrooms and spinach, then stir them into a pot of creamy gluten-free risotto made with vegetable broth.

Quinoa and Black Bean Tacos:

9. Fill gluten-free corn tortillas with a mixture of quinoa, black beans, corn, and your favorite taco toppings.

Cauliflower Steak with Chimichurri:

10. Slice cauliflower into steaks, roast until golden, and drizzle with a zesty chimichurri sauce made from herbs, garlic, and olive oil.

You are welcome to alter these recipes to suit your dietary requirements and taste preferences. Enjoy your delicious gluten-free vegan dinners!

Chapter six

Delightful Gluten-Free Vegan Snacks, Salads, and Sandwiches

Embracing a gluten-free vegan lifestyle doesn't mean sacrificing flavor or variety. Elevate your culinary experience with these delectable and nutritious snacks, salads, and sandwiches specially crafted for beginners on the gluten-free vegan journey.

Snacks

**1. Roasted Chickpeas:
Crunchy and protein-packed, roasted chickpeas seasoned with your favorite spices make for an irresistible snack. Perfect for

on-the-go munching or as a satisfying movie-night treat.

**2. Guacamole with Veggie Sticks:

Dive into a bowl of creamy guacamole paired with colorful veggie sticks. Avocado's richness meets the crunch of carrots, cucumber, and bell peppers for a guilt-free indulgence.

**3. Trail Mix Bliss:

Create your custom trail mix with a blend of gluten-free nuts, seeds, and dried fruits. This energy-boosting snack is ideal for satisfying midday cravings or fueling your outdoor adventures.

Salads

**1. Rainbow Quinoa Salad:

A vibrant medley of cooked quinoa, cherry tomatoes, cucumber, and bell peppers. Drizzle with a zesty lemon vinaigrette for a refreshing salad that bursts with color and nutrients.

**2. Kale and Mango Salad:

Massage kale leaves with a citrusy dressing, and toss with diced mango, red onion, and a sprinkle of pumpkin seeds. This nutrient-packed salad is both satisfying and delicious.

**3. Caprese Salad with a Twist:

Reimagine the classic Caprese by using gluten-free vegan mozzarella, ripe tomatoes, fresh basil, and a balsamic glaze. A simple yet sophisticated dish that captures the essence of summer.

Sandwiches

**1. Avocado and Hummus Wrap:

Spread a gluten-free tortilla with creamy avocado and hummus. Add lettuce, tomato, and your favorite veggies for a quick and satisfying wrap that's perfect for lunch or a light dinner.

**2. Grilled Vegetable Panini:

Layer grilled zucchini, eggplant, and bell peppers between two slices of gluten-free bread. Press until golden brown for a hearty and flavorful panini experience.

**3. Chickpea Salad Sandwich:

Mash chickpeas and mix with vegan mayo, celery, and spices. Pile the mixture onto

gluten-free bread with crisp lettuce for a
delightful, protein-packed sandwich.

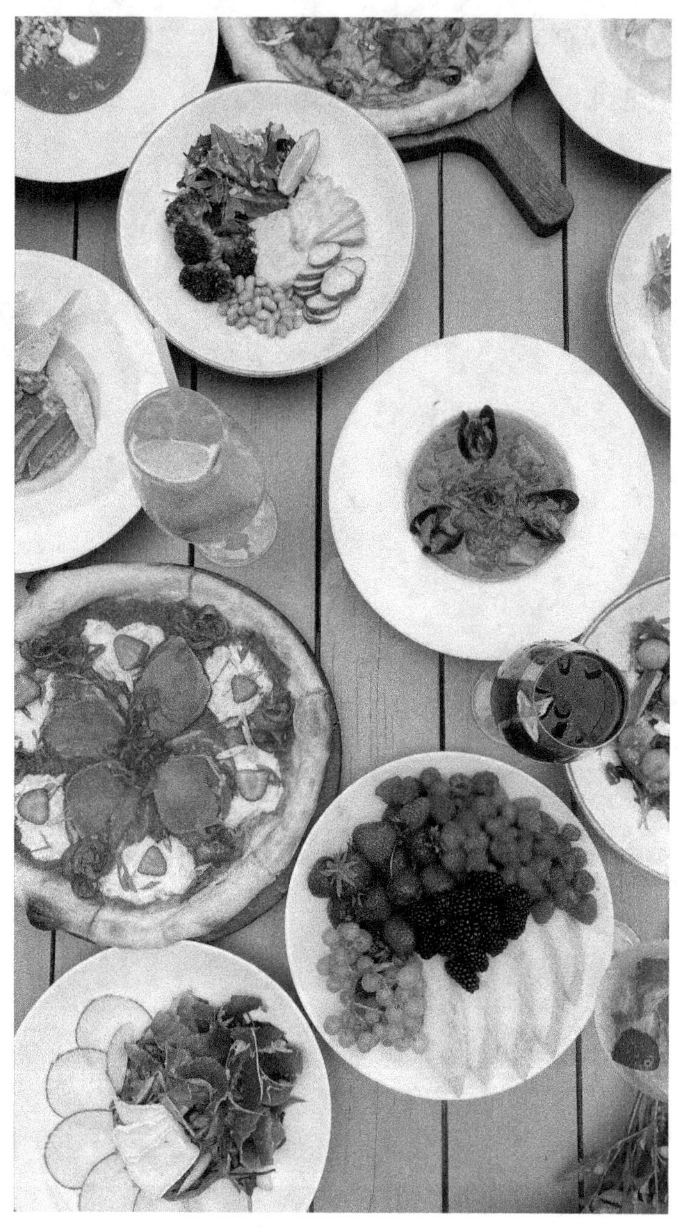

Chapter seven

Special treats and Desserts

Indulging in special treats and desserts can be a delightful experience, even for those following a gluten-free vegan lifestyle. Here are some tempting and satisfying options to sweeten your moments:

Special Treats

**1. Chocolate Avocado Mousse:

Blend ripe avocados with cocoa powder, sweetener of choice, and a splash of vanilla. This rich and creamy mousse is a decadent treat that's surprisingly healthy.

**2. Coconut Bliss Balls:

Combine shredded coconut, dates, and a touch of almond butter in a food processor. Roll into bite-sized balls for a sweet, energy-boosting snack.

**3. Dark Chocolate-Dipped Strawberries:

 Fresh strawberries should be dipped in molten dark chocolate and let to cool. This elegant yet simple treat is perfect for special occasions or a sweet pick-me-up.

Desserts

**1. Gluten-Free Vegan Brownies:

Use a gluten-free flour blend and substitute eggs with flax eggs to create fudgy and irresistible brownies. Add chopped nuts or dairy-free chocolate chips for extra indulgence.

**2. Chia Seed Pudding Parfait:

Layer chia seed pudding with fresh berries and gluten-free granola for a parfait that combines creamy, crunchy, and fruity elements.

**3. Pumpkin Spice Cupcakes:

Bake gluten-free cupcakes infused with pumpkin puree and warming spices. Top with dairy-free cream cheese frosting for a festive and delicious treat.

**4. Cinnamon-Sugar Baked Apples:

Core and slice apples, then bake with a sprinkle of cinnamon and coconut sugar until tender. Serve warm for a comforting and wholesome dessert.

**5. Berry Coconut Ice Cream:

Blend frozen berries with coconut milk and a sweetener of choice. Freeze the mixture for a few hours to create a refreshing and dairy-free ice cream.

**6. Lemon Blueberry Cheesecake Bites:

Make a gluten-free crust using almond flour and coconut oil, then layer with a cashew-based cheesecake filling swirled with fresh blueberries.

Special Treats for Children

**1. Fruit Kabobs with Chocolate Drizzle:

Skewer colorful fruits like strawberries, bananas, and pineapple. Drizzle with melted

dark chocolate for a fun and tasty treat that
kids will love.

**2. Almond Butter Rice Crispy Treats:

Replace traditional marshmallows with a
mixture of almond butter, brown rice syrup, and
gluten-free rice crisps. Shape into squares for
a healthier twist on a classic favorite.

**3. Mini Gluten-Free Vegan Donuts:

Bake bite-sized donuts using a gluten-free flour
blend. Coat with a dusting of powdered sugar
or cinnamon for a delightful, kid-friendly treat.

Desserts for Pregnant Women

**1. Avocado Chocolate Pudding:

Whip up a creamy chocolate pudding using
avocados, cocoa powder, and a natural

sweetener. Rich in healthy fats and satisfying for pregnancy cravings.

**2. Berry Bliss Smoothie Bowl:

Blend mixed berries with a banana, almond milk, and a scoop of vegan protein powder. Pour into a bowl and top with gluten-free granola for a nourishing and refreshing dessert.

**3. Sweet Potato Pie Bites:

Create bite-sized sweet potato pie treats by mixing mashed sweet potatoes with warm spices like cinnamon and nutmeg. Spoon the mixture into mini tart shells for a delightful indulgence.

All-Ages Favorites

**1. Chocolate Chip Chickpea Cookies:

Make cookies using chickpea flour, vegan chocolate chips, and coconut oil. These cookies offer a protein boost and are both kid-friendly and pregnancy-safe.

**2. Fruit Sorbet Popsicles:

Blend your favorite fruits with a bit of maple syrup, freeze in popsicle molds, and enjoy a refreshing, naturally sweetened treat suitable for all ages.

**3. Banana Ice Cream Sandwiches:

Slice bananas, spread them with peanut or almond butter, and create mini sandwiches. Freeze for a satisfying and nutritious frozen dessert.

Ensuring a balance of nutrients and flavors, these gluten-free vegan treats cater to the diverse tastes of children and the nutritional needs of pregnant women. Feel free to customize these recipes based on individual preferences and dietary requirements. Enjoy the joyous moments of savoring these special treats!

Vegans and Glute-free recipes for elderly members of home

Crafting gluten-free and vegan recipes for elderly members involves considering both nutritional needs and taste preferences. Here are some wholesome and delicious options tailored for elderly individuals:

Breakfast

**1. Quinoa Porridge with Berries:

Cook quinoa in almond milk and top with a medley of fresh berries. Add a sprinkle of chopped nuts for a nutrient-packed and easy-to-digest breakfast.

**2. Chia Seed Pudding with Mango:

Combine chia seeds with coconut milk and refrigerate overnight. Top with ripe mango slices for a delicious and fiber-rich morning treat.

Lunch

**1. Lentil and Vegetable Soup:

Prepare a hearty lentil soup with carrots, celery, and spinach. Season with herbs like thyme and rosemary for comforting and easy-to-chew nutrition.

**2. Stuffed Bell Peppers with Quinoa:

Create a soft and flavorful filling by combining quinoa with soft veggies like zucchini and tomatoes. Bake until peppers are tender for a nourishing main course.

Dinner

**1. Baked Sweet Potato with Vegan Chili:

Roast sweet potatoes and serve with a gentle vegan chili made from kidney beans, tomatoes, and spices. This dish is both comforting and easily digestible.

**2. Cauliflower and Chickpea Curry:

Prepare a mild curry using cauliflower, chickpeas, and coconut milk. Serve over basmati rice for a fragrant and gentle dinner option.

Snacks

**1. Soft Fruit Smoothies:

Blend ripe bananas with berries and a dollop of almond or soy yogurt. These smoothies provide hydration, vitamins, and a delightful snack for any time of day.

**2. Hummus with Sliced Cucumbers:

Pair homemade hummus with thinly sliced cucumbers for a light and protein-rich snack that's easy to chew.

Desserts

**1. Baked Apples with Cinnamon:

Apples should be cored, sliced, sprinkled with cinnamon, and baked until soft. Top with a dollop of dairy-free vanilla yogurt for a sweet and comforting dessert.

**2. Coconut Rice Pudding:

Simmer rice in coconut milk with a touch of sweetener. Serve warm or chilled for a soothing and gentle dessert option.

These recipes are designed to be not only flavorful but also easily digestible for elderly members. Always consider individual dietary restrictions and preferences when preparing meals.

Conclusion

In conclusion, the "30-Minute Gluten-Free Vegan Cookbook for Beginners" offers a delightful entry into the world of plant-based, gluten-free cuisine. With its emphasis on quick and accessible recipes, it empowers beginners to create delicious meals without sacrificing flavor or time. The cookbook not only addresses dietary needs but also champions the idea that a vibrant, inclusive kitchen is within reach for everyone. From innovative ingredient substitutions to time-saving cooking techniques, this cookbook proves that embracing a gluten-free and vegan lifestyle can be both convenient and delectable. It's a culinary journey where simplicity meets creativity, making it a must-have guide for those embarking on the exciting adventure of

gluten-free vegan cooking. Happy cooking!

www.ingramcontent.com/pod-product-compliance
Lightning Source LLC
Chambersburg PA
CBHW061005260726
48661CB00005B/2066